Green Smoothie Power

Boost Your Energy and Health

Table of Contents

Chapter 1. Introduction

Welcome to "Green Smoothie Power: Boost Your Energy and Health" - a special report that guides you on a flavorful journey towards wellness. Overflowing with vitality and brimming with nature's best, green smoothies are more than just a refreshing beverage – they're life-enhancers tucked away in a gleaming glass! This report isn't packed with complex terminology or intricate details. Instead, it's a vibrant, easy-to-digest guide, stirring together science, health benefits, and delicious recipes to make adding a power-packed smoothie to your routine a delight. Envision creating concoctions abundant with kale or spinach, rounding off with fruity boosts, and jazzed up with superfoods while doing wonders for your health! Unearth the secrets of harnessing nature's bounty and savor the true essence of vitality one sip at a time. Between these covers, health and flavor collide in an emerald whirlpool. Are you ready to turn a new leaf towards ultimate wellness? Let's get blending!

Chapter 2. The Power of Green: An Introduction to Green Smoothies

Green smoothies are vibrant, nutrient-dense drinks created by blending green leafy vegetables, fruits, and water. They showcase earth's incredible bounty, offering nutritionally rich ingredients that bring myriad benefits to your overall health. These refreshing beverages are renowned for their valuable nutrients, hassle-free creation process, and delightful versatility in taste.

2.1. Myth Busted: Let's Start from the Basics

If you find yourself hesitant to take your first sip of a green smoothie due to its colors or possible taste, remember that green doesn't equate to bland or bitter. Although the base is comprised of leafy greens - even the thought of which can be a turn-off for some - the inclusion of choice fruits adds a sweet and tangy facet, which balances out flavors and makes these drinks rather enjoyable.

Green smoothies are quite unlike what most people think - they're a delightful blend of taste and health, far different from the infamous nutritious-but-disgusting wellness foods. They are fabulously flexible, allowing you to experiment with a variety of ingredients. The sky is your limit when creating the ultimate green smoothie!

2.2. Worlds of Greens: Unlocking the Nutrient Powerhouses

Guarding the green in these smoothies are nutrient powerhouses such as spinach, kale, collards, celery, cucumber, etc. These vegetables act as nutritional superheroes, introducing a remarkable suite of vitamins, minerals, fibers into your diet, and promoting optimal health. Each veggie brings something unique to the table, such as: - Spinach: This leafy green is abundant in iron, potassium, and calcium - Kale: Among other vitamins, kale is a great source of vitamin K, which aids clotting and bone health - Celery: It offers a solid source of vitamin A, crucial for vision and immune function - Cucumber: This refreshing ingredient is a hydration hero, offering a hydrating base for your smoothies

2.3. Sweeten the Deal: Blend in Some Fruits

For those concerned about the possible bitter taste of greens, there's nothing to worry about. Key players like bananas, berries, mangoes, and peaches introduce natural sweetness to your smoothie, offsetting the natural "green" taste.

Let's take a quick look at their nutrient profile: - Bananas: This accessible fruit is rich in potassium and vitamin C - Berries: Regardless of the kind, berries are packed with antioxidants - Mangoes: A tropical delight loaded with vitamins A and C - Peaches: These juicy fruits provide a significant amount of vitamin A

2.4. Transformation with Health: The Health Benefits of Green Smoothies

With the promise of delivering naturally rich nutrients and antioxidants, green smoothies bring along remarkable health benefits. Regular inclusion in your diet may result in better digestion, weight loss, detoxification, improved hydration, and robust immunity. Plus, green smoothies can contribute towards a more youthful appearance, better skin, and an overall sense of well-being.

When considering your nourishment, it's worth mentioning that it's not just the sheer number of nutrients and antioxidants that matter. It's about how well our bodies can absorb and use them—a setting where green smoothies shine like no other. Blending the ingredients breaks down the hard-to-digest cellular structure of vegetables, allowing your body to maximally utilize the nutrients.

2.5. Blends of Vitality: Crafting Your Perfect Green Smoothie

Crafting a perfect green smoothie isn't an art of precise measures or rigid routines; rather, it's a vibrant play of personal tastes, needs, and whims. Green smoothies adapt wonderfully to complement your taste exactly, no matter how sweet, tart, tropical, or simple you want it to be.

In the next chapters, we will dive into the 'how-to' of creating your perfect smoothie blend, unraveling a rainbow of healthful ingredients, their benefits, and combinations that can help you greet each day with a splash of vitality.

Remember, the secret of enjoying green smoothies is not about following a particular recipe or ingredient set. It is about creating a bespoke blend that suits your taste buds and nutritional needs.

In your journey towards health and wellness, green smoothies can emerge as a trusted ally. Brimming with nature's delight, these densely packed nutritious drinks offer a refreshing leap into a healthier lifestyle, one loving sip at a time. So, are you ready to step into a world where health and taste are not conflicting territories but harmoniously mingle in a glass of endless goodness? Join the green revolution today and experience the blend of vitality!

Chapter 3. Superfuel Foods: Nutrient-rich Ingredients for Your Smoothies

Superfoods are nutritional powerhouses that pack large amounts of antioxidants, polyphenols, vitamins, and minerals. Introducing these nutrient-dense foods into your smoothies can significantly boost their health benefits. Combining green leafy vegetables, fruits, seeds, and other classified superfoods, you can create a liquid gold mine of nutrients, perfect for aiding in disease prevention, weight loss, and promoting overall vitality.

3.1. Green Leafy Vegetables

Starting your superfood journey with green leafy vegetables is an excellent place to begin. Green leafy vegetables are loaded with vitamins A, C, K, and several B vitamins. They are also an excellent source of dietary fiber, calcium, iron, and potassium.

Some of the most nutrient-dense leafy greens include:

- Kale: Considered one of the most nutrient-rich foods on the planet, kale is packed with vitamins A, C, and K. Plus, it's a good source of fiber, protein, thiamin, riboflavin, folate, iron, and manganese.

- Spinach: High in niacin, zinc, protein, fiber, vitamins A, C, E and K, thiamin, vitamin B6, folate, calcium, iron, magnesium, phosphorus, potassium, copper, and manganese.

- Swiss Chard: Rich in vitamins A, K, and C, as well as a good source of magnesium, potassium, iron, and dietary fiber.

- Collard Greens: Collard greens are loaded with vitamins A, C, and K, as well as calcium, dietary fiber, and multiple B vitamins.

Incorporating these nutritious greens into your smoothies won't only boost nutrient content but can also help enhance the smoothie's color and flavor.

3.2. Fruits: Nature's Candy

Fruits are nature's candy—sweet, flavorful, and loaded with essential nutrients. Many fruits are high in fiber and packed with antioxidants. Here are a few superfruits you might consider:

- Berries (blueberries, strawberries, raspberries): Berries are packed with an array of antioxidants, fiber, and vitamin C. They're also known for their anti-inflammatory properties.

- Bananas: A good source of potassium and vitamin C, bananas also contribute a creamy texture to smoothies.

- Apples: High in antioxidants, especially Vitamin C, and dietary fiber, apples add a natural sweetness to your concoctions.

- Oranges: Bursting with vitamin C, a potent antioxidant, oranges also provide a unique zesty flavor.

A dash of these fruits can give your green smoothie a refreshing twist, making it delicious and more palatable.

3.3. Seeds and Nuts

While green leafy vegetables and fruits generally make up the base of a green smoothie, adding seeds and nuts could elevate its nutritional value. Some notable seeds and nuts include:

- Chia Seeds: These are packed with Omega-3 fatty acids, fiber, protein, and various micronutrients.

- Hemp Seeds: These seeds are an excellent source of protein and contain all nine essential amino acids. They are also high in fat, including Omega-3 and Omega-6 fatty acids.

- Flax Seeds: A rich source of the Omega-3 fatty acid ALA, fiber, and high-quality protein.

- Almonds: High in healthy monounsaturated fats, fiber, protein, and various essential nutrients.

Seeds and nuts not only improve the nutrient profile of your smoothie but also add a satisfying crunch if sprinkled on top.

3.4. Superfoods

Superfood is a term used to describe food with high nutritional density and associated health benefits. Below are a few superfoods you can incorporate into your smoothies:

- Spirulina: A type of blue-green algae that is loaded with various nutrients, high-quality protein, and powerful antioxidants that can reduce inflammation.

- Wheatgrass: High in nutrients and antioxidants, wheatgrass is also believed to have various health benefits, such as reducing cholesterol and aiding weight loss.

- Cacao: Raw cacao is packed with antioxidants and can boost your mood and cognitive performance.

- Bee Pollen: Rich in vitamins, minerals, proteins, lipids, and fatty acids, as well as enzymes and co-enzymes. It's touted for its rejuvenating and revitalizing properties.

- Açaí Berries: High in antioxidants, fiber and heart-healthy fats, these berries can be consumed as a freeze-dried powder in smoothies.

Diving into the assortment of superfoods available, you'll find that each one offers a unique set of health benefits that can effectively boost your smoothie game.

The power of superfoods is undeniable. Infusing your green

smoothie with these nutrient-rich ingredients can significantly enhance its nutritional profile, leading to numerous health benefits. Remember that variety is key, so don't be afraid to mix and match these ingredients to create a smoothie that caters to your taste and nutritional needs. Your journey towards a healthier, more sustainable lifestyle is in your hands, or rather, in your glass. Cheers to good health!

Chapter 4. Unmasking the Health Benefits: What Makes Green Smoothies So Good

With their verdant hue and refreshing taste, green smoothies are more than just a pleasing sight or palate—you are literally taking in life-sustaining nutrients in every sip. But what exactly makes green smoothies so good? Let's bring forth the untold story of the health virtues hidden in that emerald glass.

4.1. The Power of Greens

Primarily composed of leafy greens such as spinach, kale, and collards, these smoothies serve as an easy avenue to achieve the recommended daily intake of vegetables. With them comes a wealth of phytonutrients—plant compounds that play a crucial role in maintaining optimal health.

Phytonutrients found in leafy greens boast anti-inflammatory and antioxidant properties. These aid in combating oxidative stress—a contributing factor in chronic diseases such as heart disease and different forms of cancer.

Moreover, leafy greens are rich in dietary fiber, which support a healthy digestive tract and contribute to feelings of fullness. They also help maintain healthy blood glucose and cholesterol levels.

4.2. Fruity Elevation

Fruits, another primary ingredient in green smoothies, significantly contribute to the lauded health benefits of this power-packed beverage. They not only make the smoothies tastier but also augment their nutritional profile by supplying a surplus of vitamins, minerals, and antioxidative compounds.

Vitamin C, for one, boosts the immune system and aids in maintaining the health of the skin. Fruits high in potassium, such as bananas, work in tandem with the natural sodium in your body to balance fluids and help maintain normal blood pressure.

The high fiber content in fruits also helps curb overeating by creating a feeling of satiety. And while fruits provide natural sugars, these are accompanied by fiber and thus offer a healthier alternative to processed sugars, keeping your energy steady and curb cravings.

4.3. Blend the Goodness of Superfoods

Superfoods are nutrient powerhouses that pack large doses of antioxidants, polyphenols, vitamins, and minerals. Including superfoods in your green smoothie not only enhances its health benefits but also ensures a variety of nutrients that cater to comprehensive wellbeing.

These power performers range from flaxseeds, chia seeds, spirulina to berries. They offer an array of health benefits, such as boosting the immune system, improving digestive health, reducing inflammation, and stress, and even aiding in weight loss.

4.4. Enhanced Absorption

Blending the components of a green smoothie helps break down the food particles, thus making it easier for the body to absorb the nutrients. This means you get an instant nutrient boost just from drinking your greens!

This kind of nutrient absorption is especially helpful for those who have medical conditions that can impact optimal digestion and absorption, such as Crohn's disease or irritable bowel syndrome.

4.5. Hydration and Detoxification

Green smoothies also play an important role in body detoxification. The high fiber content aids in regular bowel movement, thereby promoting the excretion of toxins. Certain fruits like apple, beetroot, and ginger are known for their detoxifying properties, thus they make an excellent addition to your smoothie.

Moreover, consuming green smoothies can contribute to your daily fluid intake, keeping you hydrated. Adequate hydration is crucial for maintaining bodily functions, skin health, and energy levels, among others.

4.6. Weight Management

Consuming green smoothies can be an effective strategy for weight management. They are low in calories yet high in nutrients and fiber, thereby promoting feelings of fullness. By adding green smoothies to your diet, you provide your body with the nourishment it needs without overloading on calories.

As a substitution for high-calorie meals or snacks, green smoothies can contribute to a healthier, controlled intake of food. It should be noted, however, that they should be consumed as part of a balanced and varied diet.

In every texture, every sip, and every ingredient in a green smoothie, nature's best is truly captured. These smoothies epitomize the harmonious blending of health and flavor, creating a refreshing taste of well-being. Understanding these health benefits will enable you to make informed decisions about what goes into your smoothie and empower you to prioritize your health. Remember, your glass of green smoothie is not just another drink—it's a testament of your commitment to wellness. Now, who's ready for another round of blending?

Chapter 5. The Energy Manifesto: Boosting Your Vitality with Green

Implementing green smoothies into your everyday schedule might seem like a challenge, but once you grasp the underlying principles and the energy-boosting effects they bring, there will be no looking back.

5.1. A Peek into Green Smoothies

Green smoothies are bursting with mineral-rich green vegetables, whole fruits, and sometimes even additional protein sources. They are loaded with phytonutrients, antioxidants, vitamins, and minerals. The primary color comes from the chlorophyll present in the leafy greens, a sturdy pigment associated with a plethora of health benefits. Think of green smoothies as a concentrated, liquid form of fruits and veggies, a beverage that can be quickly and easily absorbed by your body.

5.2. Discover the Power of Chlorophyll

Chlorophyll performs different functions inside the human body. It aids in restoring and rejuvenating our red blood cells, enhances the immune system, and helps detoxify the body by attaching to heavy metals and aiding their removal. Chlorophyll is also renowned for its alkalizing properties and aids in maintaining our body's pH levels, an essential aspect of human health.

5.3. How Green Smoothies Boost Energy

The main reason green smoothies are such an excellent energy resource has much to do with their digestion process. They are high in fiber, which aids in digestion, and keeps our gut flora healthy, resulting in an energy boost. By merging our greens with fruits, we allow the fruit's natural sugars to propel our energy levels upwards immediately. Meanwhile, the robust fibrous content of green vegetables prolongs this energy boost keeping us satisfied and invigorated over an extended period.

5.4. The Green Vegetables for Power-Packed Smoothies

While it might be tempting to add a variety of vegetables to your mix, the backbone to a great green smoothie is usually a leafy green vegetable. Here are some primary contenders:

1. Spinach: Packed with vitamins A, K, and essential minerals like iron and manganese, spinach is an all-around superfood that's mild enough not to dominate the taste of your smoothie.

2. Kale: This leafy green brings a pack of vitamin C, K, and a suite of B vitamins. It's also a great plant-based source of calcium.

3. Chard: Along with having ample amounts of vitamin K, chard has a unique combo of nutrients that makes it excellent for controlling blood sugars.

5.5. Fruity Exuberance: The Perfect Complement

Fruits not only add pops of flavor but also provide a natural sweetness to our smoothies. They are also responsible for the immediate energy boost due to their natural sugar content. Here are some fruit options:

1. Berries: Strawberries, blueberries, raspberries, and blackberries are high in antioxidants and lend wonderful flavors to your fusion.

2. Bananas: These add creaminess to your blend while offering potassium and vitamin B6. They're also an excellent source of quick energy due to their carbohydrate content.

3. Pineapple: Besides its tropical flair, pineapple offers digestive enzymes, making it a unique fruit choice for smoothies.

5.6. Integration into Daily Routine

Integrating green smoothies into your daily routine doesn't necessarily mean a total dietary shift. It's about making subtle changes to your pattern of eating. A green smoothie can replace one of your snacks, or better yet, kickstart your day with one. They make for an excellent energy source in the morning or a perfect mid-afternoon pick-me-up, ensuring you can ward off any fatigue and stay productive.

5.7. Intricate Blending Equals Enhanced Nutrition

Blending breaks down the cell walls of fruits and vegetables, consequently making it easier for the body to access and absorb nutrients. When blended well, the cell walls within the fruits and vegetables open and expose digestive enzymes to a more comprehensive range of nutritional benefits.

5.8. Make Most of Your Greens

While green smoothies can undoubtedly boost your energy levels and greatly benefit your health, drinking the same smoothie every day might limit the range of nutrients you take in. Therefore, rotating your greens and varying your ingredients can ensure you're receiving a broad spectrum of nutrients and vitamins.

Savory and healthful, green smoothies are nothing short of a culinary triumph. With just a blender, some fresh produce, and the knowledge outlined in this chapter, you could be a step closer towards superior wellness and vitality. Savor the power of green and unlock a fresh dimension of health – one sip at a time.

Chapter 6. Green Smoothie Recipes for Beginners: Your Kickstart Guide

Dipping your toes into the world of green smoothies can seem a bit daunting at first. Suddenly, you have to think about which fruits marry best with which vegetables, whether to throw in some protein powder or a handful of chia seeds, and much more. But fret not! This guide will gradually guide you through the process, ensuring you become a green smoothie expert in no time.

6.1. The Green Smoothie Blueprint

A well-rounded green smoothie typically consists of 40% greens and 60% fruits. Add-ins such as seeds, nuts, herbs, and spices offer an extra boost of nutrition and flavor. Here's a simple blueprint to make your own green concoction:

1. ingredients

Greens

Fruits

Add-Ins

Spinach

Bananas

Flaxseeds

Kale

Mangoes

Chia Seeds

Swiss Chard

Berries

Ginger

Romaine Lettuce

Oranges

Cacao Powder

Choose one ingredient from each column and blend away. The beauty of a green smoothie is in its versatility! You can mix and match according to your preference.

6.2. Beginner-Friendly Green Smoothie Recipes

Let's start gently, captivating your palette with simple, delightful flavors. Here are a few beginner-friendly green smoothie recipes to kickstart your journey to wellness.

1. **Banana-Orange-Ginger Smoothie**

You'll Need: * 2 cups of spinach * 1 banana * 1 orange, peeled * 1 teaspoon of grated ginger * 1 cup of water

Peel and dice the fruits if necessary. Blend spinach and water until smooth. Add fruits and ginger into the blender. Blend again until smooth, pour into a glass and enjoy.

1. **Mango-Berry Blast Smoothie**

You'll Need: * 2 cups of kale, stems removed * 1 cup of frozen mango * 1 cup of mixed berries * 1 cup of almond milk

Blend the kale and almond milk until smooth. Add the fruits, blend again until smooth, then serve. The almond milk lends this smoothie a creamy touch, while the frozen fruits keep it thick and chilled.

1. **Tropical Green Delight Smoothie**

You'll Need: * 2 cups of swiss chard, stems removed * 1 cup of frozen pineapple * 1 cup of frozen kiwi * 1 cup of coconut water

Begin by blending the swiss chard and coconut water. Follow up with the fruits, blend again until smooth, and end this mild tropical adventure with a delightful sip.

6.3. Customizing Your Green Smoothie

While sticking to recipes is a good start, customizing your smoothie to suit your own preferences is where things really get fun! Below, we'll guide you on how to tweak the texture, flavor, and nutritional value of your green smoothie.

1. **A Dash of Creaminess**: Adding 1/4 to 1/2 an avocado, a scoop of Greek yogurt, or a tablespoon of nut butter can provide a wonderfully creamy consistency to your smoothie.

2. **Natural Sweetness**: If you prefer your smoothie a bit sweeter, consider adding naturally sweet fruits like ripe bananas, mangoes, apples, or pears. You can also add a spoonful of raw honey, maple syrup, or soaked dried dates.

3. **Protein Boost**: To turn your smoothie into a fuller meal, consider adding protein-rich foods such as Greek yogurt, protein powder, silken tofu, or nut butter.

6.4. Dos and Don'ts for Your Green Smoothie

Remember, your green smoothie journey is a marathon, not a sprint. Here, we outline some useful dos and don'ts that will keep things tasty and enjoyable.

DO's

- Do add liquids first: Always add your liquid first to ensure smooth blending.

- Do rotate your greens: To prevent buildup of oxalic acid.

- Do experiment: Have fun with your ingredients and try something new each time!

DON'Ts

- Don't overload on sweet fruits: Green smoothies should be a balance of fruits and veggies.

- Don't neglect the fiber: Fiber aids digestion and gives you a sense of satiety.

With this comprehensive guide, you are now equipped to create luscious green concoctions that fuel your body with nature's best. The prospect of your wellness journey may seem intensive but it's absolutely worthwhile - after all, your health is at stake. Eventually, you won't just be blending fruits and veggies - you'll be blending your way to a healthier, more vibrant you. Happy blending!

Chapter 7. Advanced Blends: Recipes for the Seasoned Smoothie Lover

You've embarked on a verdant voyage through the world of green smoothies, unraveling the power of nature's most nutrient-dense offerings, and applying them in your day-to-day diet. Now, you're no longer a green beginner. You've mastered the basics and you're ready for the next challenge— creating advanced blends teeming with diverse flavors and potent health benefits.

7.1. The Uncharted Territory of Advanced Blending

In this new stage of your green smoothie journey, you'll be experimenting with different ingredients, embracing a variety of flavors from sweet to savory, and reaping the amazing benefits of potent superfoods. As a seasoned smoothie lover, you'll need a wider array of ingredients and a more sophisticated palate to appreciate the complex flavors.

Remember, these advanced blends are about more than just tossing greens into a blender. They involve pairing and layering ingredients for maximum flavor and nutritional content. Using a high-quality blender will help you create smoother textures and extract the maximum nutrients from your ingredients.

7.2. The Art of Crafting Advanced Blends

Creating advanced blends does not mean you are turning your back on the basics. In many ways, they still bear the hallmarks of your beginner's green smoothie, with greens, fruits, and liquids making up the base. But let's turn it up a notch. This section will focus on special ingredients we seldom use and would often overlook but are excellent in delivering unique flavors and remarkable health benefits.

1. *Sea Greens* – Underwater vegetables like spirulina, kelp, and dulse are loaded with minerals. They reinforce our thyroid function and are wonderful at detoxification.

2. *Fermented Foods* – Kefir, yoghurt, or kombucha added to your smoothie will infuse it with natural probiotics, boosting your gut health and fortifying your immune system.

3. *Exotic Fruits* – Add fruits like dragon fruit, lychee, or papaya to give your green smoothie a tropical flair. These fruits are packed with unique antioxidants and digestive enzymes.

4. *Herbs and Spices* – Turmeric, cinnamon, ginger, or basil can introduce exciting flavors and come with their own health benefits, like increasing metabolic rates and reducing inflammation.

5. *Healthy Fats* – Don't be afraid of adding in some unprocessed healthy fats like avocado, nut butter, or flaxseeds, which will make your shake more satisfying and offer essential fatty acids.

7.3. Exhilarating Advanced Blends Recipes

The following recipes demonstrate the potential to experiment with flavors and nutritional profiles. They not only taste fantastic, but each blend offers compelling health benefits.

- *Thyroid Tonic*
    - 1 cup of coconut water

- 1 banana, peeled

- 1 cup of blueberries, fresh or frozen

- 2 cups of spinach

- 1 tablespoon of spirulina Blend all the ingredients and enjoy cold. It's a thyroid-friendly potion that aids in detoxification.

- *Tropical Gut Soother*

  - 1 cup of almond milk

  - 1 cup of coconut yoghurt

  - 1 large papaya, peeled

  - 1/2 cup of pineapple chunks

  - 1 Tbsp of chia seeds Begin by blending the almond milk and yoghurt, then add the fruits and finally the chia seeds. This recipe is ideal for healing the gut and imparting a tropical vibe.

- *Metabolic Magic*

  - 1 cup of chilled green tea

  - 1 handful of kale

  - 1 apple, cored

  - 1 carrot, peeled

  - 1 tablespoon of ginger, grated Blend all ingredients until smooth, starting with the green tea and ending with ginger. This shake helps to kick-start your metabolism thanks to the capsaicin in ginger.

7.4. Powering Up Your Blends with Superfoods

Superfoods are powerful, concentrated sources of nutrients that can transform your smoothies into ultra-nourishing meals. Here are the top five superfoods to add to your advanced blends:

1. *Chia Seeds* – They are high in Omega-3 fatty acids, fiber, and protein. They add a creamy texture to your smoothie as they absorb the liquid, resulting in a satiating, meal-like drink.

2. *Hemp Seeds* – They offer protein and the perfect balance of Omega-3 to Omega-6 fatty acids. They have a nutty flavor that complements green smoothies well.

3. *Moringa* – This leafy green is absolutely packed with protein, antioxidants, and electrolytes. It has a mildly sweet, grassy flavor that blends seamlessly into smoothies.

4. *Cacao* – Rich in magnesium, iron, and antioxidants, cacao can transform your smoothie into a healthy and fitting dessert.

5. *Maca* – It works as an adaptogen, helping your body deal with stress. It has a malty flavor and can give your smoothie a delicious energy boost.

As an advanced smoothie maker, you have the potential to make every glass a creative, health-boosting blend. Experiment, enjoy, and let the greens guide you to greater health and vitality. Just remember, quantity doesn't trump quality when it comes to ingredients—choose fresh, organic products whenever possible. With this guide, you're one step closer to the ultimate wellness you're seeking. Good luck, and happy blending!

Chapter 8. Beyond the Glass: Incorporating Green Smoothies into Your Daily Diet

Adopting the green smoothie lifestyle is a big step towards holistic health and wellness. Adding a glass of green smoothie into your daily diet is not just about blending in some greens and fruits. It's a commitment - a promise to yourself to lead a healthier, more vibrant life. Once you start with this habit, it significantly transforms how you perceive nutrition, blending it seamlessly with taste.

8.1. The Elixir of Life: Understanding the Power of Green Smoothies

Green smoothies are an exceptional source of natural vitamins and minerals, procured primarily from fresh greens including spinach, kale, celery, cucumber, and other leafy greens. These are combined with juicy fruits like apples, pears, bananas, and berries to make it flavorful. The addition of superfoods like chia seeds, flax seeds or spirulina heighten their health quotient. This potpourri of fiber, antioxidants, essential nutrients, and plant-based proteins positions green smoothies as a power-packed meal substitute or a snack.

8.2. Trailblazing a Healthy Morning Tradition

Start your day with a jolt of nutrition by amalgamating a green smoothie into your breakfast routine. It's as simple as blending a handful of leafy greens, a portion of fruits, and a teaspoon of superfood with your preferred liquid base like water, coconut water, or almond milk. This 5-minute recipe can be prepped the night before. All you need to do is blend it and savor it first thing in the morning.

8.3. Complement Your Meals with Vitality

In addition to breaking your fast, green smoothies can be a nutritional addition to your meals. Pair it alongside your lunch to reap double the benefits. Opt for recipes with a lighter flavor profile that won't overshadow your main course. The midday replenishment of crucial vitamins and minerals will provide sustained energy for the remainder of the day.

8.4. Bridge the Nutritional Gap with a Midday Smoothie Snack

Late afternoon lulls often send us reaching for caffeine or sugary snacks. A simple solution - replace those unhealthy options with a green smoothie packed with energy-boosting nutrients. Select fruits like bananas or oranges that naturally supplement the energy you need while keeping you satiated until the next meal.

8.5. Green Nights: Ease Your Night Time Cravings

Looking for a post-dinner guilt-free dessert? A green smoothie made with fruits like pineapples, mangoes or berries and a generous dollop of Greek yogurt, provides a creamy, dessert-like texture while keeping your calorie count in check.

8.6. Customization: The Key to Consistency

Boredom can often deter your transformation to a healthier lifestyle. To ensure you stay on track, try altering ingredients and experimenting with different combinations of greens, fruits, nuts, and seeds. Personalize your smoothie by adding non-dairy milk, plant-based protein powders, or a pinch of spices like turmeric or ginger.

8.7. The Budget-Friendly Health Booster

Green smoothies are an affordable way to pump nutrients into your diet. With the basic ingredients being fruits and vegetables, you can create a vibrant smoothie bowl without digging a hole in your pocket. Opt for seasonal produce, buy in bulk, and freeze for future use.

8.8. Harnessing the Green Advantage in Special Diets

Whether you are gluten free, vegan, paleo, or following a low carb diet - green smoothies can easily be tailored to fit your dietary needs. For a low carb version, simply select low sugar fruits like green apples or strawberries. For protein-packed smoothies, include your favorite vegan protein powder or nut butter.

Incorporating green smoothies into your diet is much more than a dietary change. It's about embracing a journey towards improved wellness. With each glass, you consume the power of nature - potent, serene and full of life. Each sip brings you closer to a healthier version of yourself, paving the way to enhanced vitality, radiant lifelong health, and an overall sense of wellbeing.

Follow this guide diligently, adapt it to your unique requirements, and soon you will notice the positive changes reverberating through your lifestyle. Remember, the goal is not just to live but to thrive, and green smoothies are certainly your perfect partner in this journey. Are you ready to blend your way to better health?

Chapter 9. Kid-friendly Concoctions: Initiating the Little Ones into the Green Revolution

Many adults find the prospect of drinking a beverage that's green, let alone convincing children to do the same, a daunting task. However, with the increasing awareness about health and wellness, it's become necessary to introduce children to healthier lifestyle choices, one sip at a time. The journey starts right here, by initiating the little ones into the green revolution with a range of kid-friendly green smoothie concoctions.

9.1. The Green Gateway

Before diving into the world of green smoothies, it's vital to understand their significance. They're nature's blend of vegetables, fruits, nuts, and seeds, juiced or blended together in perfect harmony. Primarily, green smoothies are excellent sources of vitamins, minerals, fiber, and other essential nutrients. But, more than just their nutritional aspect, these drinks serve as a wonderful way to introduce children to an array of fruits and vegetables that they might otherwise avoid. These smoothies pave the way towards healthier habits, flavors, and food choices.

9.2. Transitioning to Green

Starting the green journey doesn't mean we go all out in one swoop. Gradual introduction and an understanding of their palate are key. Begin the smoothies saga with sweeter fruits like bananas and strawberries, blended seamlessly with milder greens like baby spinach. Once they develop a liking for this, slowly and tactfully modify the spinach-to-fruit ratio, enhancing the green component step-by-step.

9.3. Fun with Flavors

Children are naturally attracted to vibrant flavors that pique their taste buds. Spice up your smoothies with natural sweeteners like honey, a dash of cinnamon or vanilla extract. These exciting flavors mask the blandness of the greens while retaining the essential nutrition. Introduce an element of surprise in their smoothie journey with unexpected but delightful additions like unsweetened cocoa powder or a hint of mint.

9.4. Smoothie Recipes

Let's delve into some basic recipes that are sure to win over the little ones:

1. **Strawberry Spinach Smoothie**

Ingredients: - 1 cup fresh spinach - 1 cup strawberries - 1 ripe banana - 1 cup almond milk - 1 tablespoon honey

Blend all ingredients until smooth, and serve chilled!

1. **Green Grapes Smoothie**

Ingredients: - 1 cup green grapes - 1 ripe banana - 1 small avocado - 1 cup coconut water - A dash of cinnamon

Combine all items in a blender and serve immediately with ice, if desired.

9.5. Engage and Involve

Children are often more inclined to consume something they've helped prepare. Involve them in the process - let them press the blender buttons, pour the smoothie into glasses, or even garnish their drink with a cherry. This involvement makes the smoothie adventure more fun and exciting.

9.6. Magical Texture

A child's sensory experience plays a significant role in their acceptance of foods. Incorporate a variety of textures by utilizing different ingredients - like chia seeds for a bit of crunch or yogurt for a creamy texture - that can enhance the smoothie's appeal.

9.7. Taking the Green a Notch up

Once the children have acquired a taste for the basic smoothie, it's time to introduce a wider greens' spectrum. Opt for kale, cucumber, or celery, but always remember the rule of thumb to start small and increase gradually.

9.8. Storytelling and Presentation

A well-narrated tale or an interesting backstory can significantly influence a child's interest in a meal. Involve colorful characters that love green smoothies, or come up with funny names for each concoction. A visually appealing presentation, such as a fun straw or a novelty cup, can also increase the smoothie's acceptability.

9.9. Beyond Greens

While green smoothies are an excellent nutritious addition to their diet, ensure it isn't the only healthy food they consume. Encourage a well-rounded diet with a mix of whole grains, fresh fruits, proteins, and other vegetables.

Once children conquer the green mountain, the rest of the wellness journey eases up. They'll grow an innate understanding of healthy eating habits, broaden their palette, and make better dietary choices in the future. As the saying goes, "Good habits formed at youth make all the difference," and this smoothie endeavor is a step in the right direction towards a healthier, greener future!

Chapter 10. Tips and Tricks: Getting the Most Out of Your Smoothie-making Routine

Commencing your green smoothie journey involves more than just tossing a few ingredients into a blender and whirling them about. For the best consistency, flavor, and health value, you need some strategic know-how. So here we go!

10.1. Quality Over Quantity

Beginning with your primary ingredients, the greens, always opt for top-notch, fresh produce. The quality and freshness of your raw materials have a significant impact on the nutrient density of your smoothie. If possible, select organic and locally grown vegetables, with no traces of harmful chemicals or pesticides.

When it comes to fruits, choose ripened ones for enhanced flavor but avoid overripe fruits, which may harbor molds and bacteria that harm your gut microbiome. However, for those necessary sub-zero icy thrills, use frozen fruits. They not only offer that sought-after chilled smoothie allure, but also solve the storage problems associated with rapid fruit spoilage.

10.2. Get That Perfect Blend

One common error is throwing every single ingredient into the blender all at once. This usually leads to an uneven blend, with hearty kale leaves remaining in chunks while fruits get almost liquefied. Instead, blend your greens with a liquid base first until they reach a smooth consistency, and then add your fruits, veggies, and boosters.

The ideal liquid base can vary depending on your personal preference and diet. You can use plain water, almond milk, coconut water, or any other non-dairy alternatives. Aim for a 60/40 ratio of fruits to greens, to keep sugars in check and make the most of the energizing power of leafy greens.

10.3. Rotate Your Greens

To ensure you're getting a broad spectrum of nutrients, it's essential to rotate your greens. Different plant classes offer diverse nutrient profiles, and alternating types of greens can help prevent developing alkaloid buildup, which some plants produce as a natural defense mechanism.

For instance, you could use spinach for a couple of days, then switch to kale or chard, followed by some romaine. This way, you'll replenish your body with a plethora of vitamins, minerals, and antioxidants.

10.4. Optimize Nutrient Absorption

A treasured tip for extracting the maximum nutritional value from your green smoothies involves adding a hint of healthy fats. Monounsaturated fats (found in foods like avocados, seeds, and nuts) can help your body absorb more phytonutrients - the compounds that give your smoothie its vibrant green color.

Another ingredient that can enhance nutritional absorption is lemon. It not only adds a zesty dimension to your smoothie but also helps in iron absorption, especially from spinach and other iron-rich greens.

10.5. Sweetening the Deal

While the fructose in fruit can sweeten your smoothies naturally, sometimes your blend might need an extra hint of sweetness. Refined sugars, artificial sweeteners, or high fructose corn syrup can sabotage the health benefits of your smoothie. Opt instead for natural sweeteners like dates, raw honey, coconut sugar, or pure maple syrup. Use these sparingly; remember, the purpose is to embrace the natural flavor of the greens and fruits.

10.6. Embrace Superfood Boosters

For that added health kick, supercharge your smoothies with superfoods. Chia seeds, goji berries, cacao nibs, spirulina, and hemp seeds are just a few nutrient-dense additions that can make your beverage from good to grand. But remember, less is more with these. A small amount can give you quite the nutrition boost without overpowering the smoothie flavor.

10.7. Mindful Consumption

Downing a massive green smoothie in mere seconds can leave you feeling bloated and full. Instead, sip it slowly, treating it as a meal rather than a quick beverage. This will allow your digestive enzymes to kick into action, breaking down the nutrients for efficient absorption.

10.8. Clean Immediately

Finally, once you've enjoyed your tasty green concoction, make a habit of cleaning your blender immediately. Leaving remnants can harden, making the cleaning process more tedious later. Plus, prompt cleaning will help prevent the growth of possible harmful bacteria while prolonging the life of your blender.

In conclusion, introducing green smoothies to your diet is an enjoyable and revolutionary step towards enhanced health. The key lies in understanding and adopting these simple yet effective tips and tricks to elevate your everyday smoothie-making routine. With them, you'll craft and savor delectable, indulgent beverages overflowing with health and vitality. Happy blending, everyone!

Chapter 11. Sustain the Change: A How-to for Green Smoothie Lifestyle Adaptation

Embracing a green smoothie lifestyle isn't about a one-off detox or a fleeting weight-loss regimen. It's about incorporating wholesome, nutritious, and delicious concoctions into your everyday life for long-lasting health benefits. Maintaining this change, however, does require a gradual acclimatization. Here, we'll walk you through the steps towards sustainability and help you adapt to living a greener, healthier lifestyle.

11.1. Understand the Benefits:

The first step towards adopting any lifestyle change is understanding why you're doing it. Green smoothies, apart from being delicious, provide an array of health bonuses. Packed with vitamins, minerals, and fiber, these nutrient-dense beverages aid in digestion, boost your immune system, improve skin health, and elevate energy levels. They also facilitate weight management by curbing unhealthy cravings and promoting a sense of fullness.

11.2. Start Small:

If you're new to the world of green smoothies, start by blending fruits with a small amount of your chosen greens. Modify the ratio slowly until your taste buds get used to the flavor, texture, and freshness of green smoothies. Gradual change allows seamless assimilation into your lifestyle.

11.3. Set Your Routine:

Identify a convenient time in your day to blend your green smoothie. This could be in the morning for a refreshing breakfast or as an energy-boosting snack in the late afternoon. Consistency is key here - once it becomes a regular part of your routine, it will seem unbearable to miss.

11.4. Variety is the Spice of Life:

Rotate your greens such as spinach, kale, collard greens, and lettuce, to keep the flavors interesting and prevent "green fatigue". Similarly, explore a range of fruits and superfoods for an enjoyable twist in your smoothies. Experimentation not only adds a layer of fun but also ensures a broad spectrum of nutrients.

11.5. Incorporate Superfoods:

Superfoods can turbocharge your green smoothies with extra nutrients. Chia seeds, flaxseeds, hemp seeds, and raw nuts offer a healthy dose of omega-3 fatty acids and proteins. Berries, like goji and acai, pack an antioxidant punch, while cacao nibs add a bite with benefits.

11.6. Plan Ahead:

To simplify your green smoothie prep, plan your blends ahead. Organize your fridge with measured bags of pre-washed greens, chopped fruits, and add-ons. You might consider prepping a week's worth of smoothies and freezing them. Simply pull out a bag and blend when it's time.

11.7. Aim for Organic:

When possible, opt for organic produce to limit exposure to pesticides and GMOs. If budget constraints are a hurdle, follow the "Dirty Dozen and Clean Fifteen" rule. Select organic for those in the Dirty Dozen (like strawberries, spinach, and kale) and go conventional for the Clean Fifteen (like avocados, pineapples, and onions).

Chapter 12. Enjoy the Journey:

Adopting a green smoothie lifestyle should be enjoyable rather than a trial. If a smoothie doesn't taste good, experiment with different ingredients until you find a blend to relish. Remember, it's a personal journey towards better health, and the best approach is always one that you can sustain.

12.1. Have a Support Network:

Sharing the journey with a like-minded individual or a group can make the adaptation process less challenging and enormously enjoyable. Having a support network to exchange recipes, share progress, and overcome plateaus can be highly motivating.

12.2. Listen to Your Body:

Above all, be in tune with your body. It's okay if your body takes time to adjust to this new dietary addition. Perhaps large quantities of greens don't sit well with you, or you might prefer consuming your green smoothie for lunch rather than breakfast. Adapt the process to fit your comfort and benefit.

12.3. The Ultimate Aim:

The primary goal is to find that perfect blend of great taste, satisfaction, and health benefits unique to your lifestyle and preferences. It's a personal experience, a journey of discovery that paves the way to a healthier, more energized version of you.

Venturing into a green smoothie lifestyle invites us into a world brimming with nutrients and flavors. With the right approach and motivations, this life-enhancing habit will sustainably integrate into your daily routine, making your health ambitions manageable, delicious, and enjoyable.